Book 1
Nutrition

By: Bring On Fitness

&

Book 2
Meal Planning

By: Bring On Fitness

&

Book 3
Weight Loss

By: Bring On Fitness

Book 1
Nutrition

The Beginners' Guide to Nutrition

By

Bring On Fitness

© Copyright 2018 – Bring On Fitness – All rights reserved.

The contents of this book may not be reproduced, duplicated, or transmitted without direct written permission from the author.

Under no circumstances will any legal responsibility or blame be held against the publisher for any reparation, damages, or monetary loss due to the information herein, either directly or indirectly.

Legal Notice:

This book is copyright protected. This is only for personal use. You cannot amend, distribute, sell, use, quote, or paraphrase any part or the content of this book without the consent of the author.

Disclaimer Notice:

Please note the information contained in this document is for educational and entertainment purposes only. Every attempt has been made to provide accurate, up-to-date, complete, and reliable information. No warranties of any kind are expressed or implied. Readers acknowledge that the author is not engaging in the rendering of legal, financial, medical, or professional advice. The content of this book has been derived from various sources. Please consult a licensed professional before attempting any techniques outlined in this book.

By reading this document, the reader agrees that under no circumstances is the author responsible for any losses, direct or indirect, which are incurred as a result of the use of

information contained within this document, including, but
not limited to, errors, omissions, or inaccuracies.

About Bring On Fitness

Our passion for fitness gave life to **Bring On Fitness**. We started with the goal of helping as many people as we can. To educate, motivate and to help change peoples lives for the better. Bring On Fitness is not only for the fitness enthusiasts, but also for the beginner. We strongly believe nothing is more important than learning the basics and creating a strong foundation in both nutrition - through meal planning, and in exercise - by following a specific plan. This is just as important for the beginner, as it is for the experienced athlete.

We set high standards for ourselves, the information we share, and the products we carry. Our goal is to provide you with exceptional products that suit your needs and the knowledge and motivation to help you work towards and achieve your health and fitness goals.

Check us out at www.bringonfitness.com

"Our Mission is to have a positive impact in changing peoples lives. We will deliver the best possible fitness and nutrition solutions that will empower people to achieve their health and fitness goals."

Table of Contents

Introduction

Nutrition matters a lot – what you put in your body is what determines your health and even how you look. It doesn't matter if you're already fit or are just trying to lose weight; knowing what you're putting into your body and how it impacts you is essential to understanding your anatomy.

Nutrition is simply about eating the right foods and avoiding those that harm you in the long term. In this book, we're going to talk about what exactly are the different components in your food. We will look at how components, such as fats, carbs, and proteins, help your body and in what proportion should you eat them. You'll also get to know what kinds of food are the best sources for these macronutrients and what kinds of food you should avoid.

A whole chapter has been dedicated to studying calories – what calories are, how they react with your body, and what their function is. Calories are essential, especially from a weight loss point of view. If you have ever tried to lose weight, the first advice you will get is how to calculate your daily calorie needs. This book will give you a brief understanding of how calories determine your weight and how you can calculate your daily calorie needs.

We are also going to look at what good fats are and the importance of lean protein in your life. Lastly, we're going to focus on the different kinds of food and drinks that anybody who wishes to be healthy should avoid.

So, if you're looking for a book that helps you understand nutrition in detail and what you should eat and in what quantity, this is the book for you.

Chapter One: Overview of Nutrition

Our bodies are not simple, and they require a lot of nutrients to function properly. Our complex structure means that different kinds of nutrition fuel different parts of our body. So if you want to survive and function correctly, you have to work on your nutritional needs.

The composition of our diet can be divided into two major groups: macronutrients and micronutrients. Together, these make up most of our nutritional needs and help us survive.

Macronutrients

There are three macronutrients, and all of them perform a specific role in helping your body absorb energy. The only function that these three nutrients perform is supplying the body with energy, and this is why you need them in high amounts so that you can repair, develop, and grow.

The three macronutrients are carbohydrates, fats, and proteins. The best thing about macronutrients is that every food item that you eat will consist of at least one of these items. Even if it's a healthy snack bar or a raw vegetable, all kinds of food are made up of these nutrients.

Fats

Fats have a lot of stigmas attached to them and are considered to be harmful. In reality, you don't have to be scared of fats at all – they are an important part of any diet, and at least 15% to 20% of what you eat should have fats.

The main purpose of fats is that they help your brain to develop, enhance the functioning of your cells, protect different parts of your body (especially organs), and help your body absorb vitamins from the food that you eat.

As fats have more than twice the amount of calories as carbohydrates and protein, they are more difficult to burn off. Therefore, fats should be consumed sparingly.

The body breaks down fats into fatty acids, which are burned as energy. Fatty acids make a fantastic energy source for the body, although it is important to note that not all cells can use fatty acids for energy; brain cells, for example, do require glucose, so be careful when thinking about limiting your carbohydrate intake. If more fatty acids are broken down than the body needs for energy at that moment, then the fatty acids are packaged together in bundles called triglycerides and then stored in fat cells for use at a later date.

Some examples of healthy fats include olives, seeds (pumpkin, chia), avocados, almonds, and walnuts.

Protein

Proteins help your cells and body tissues regrow, and they also help repair them in case they are torn. You also need proteins to have a healthy immune system and achieve hormonal balance. Proteins also have amino acids, and these are essential for your body to release hormones. Out of the 20 amino acids that are found in proteins, nine are essential for the body.

Proteins are broken down into amino acids, which are used by the body to build new proteins. Each of these proteins has a specific function, such as enabling chemical reactions or allowing cells to communicate. If the body is low in glucose and fatty acids, then the body can get energy from protein, but this is not ideal.

The right sources of protein are seeds (hemp, flax, and chia), quinoa, avocados, beets, beans, pulses and legumes, raw greens (spinach and kale), and nuts (unsalted).

Carbohydrates

Carbohydrates consist of small sugar chains, which are broken down by your digestive system and converted into glucose – the body's primary source of energy. Carbohydrates should make up at least 45% to 65% of your food consumption.

Carbohydrates, when broken down by the body into glucose, are then absorbed through the walls of the small intestine. The liver processes the glucose. It then enters the body's circulatory system, increasing the body's blood glucose levels.

This provides the body with an excellent (and quickly accessed) source of energy. If there is excess glucose, the liver will store it to be used between mealtimes if the blood glucose levels fall below a certain level.

For individuals who are starting an active lifestyle and trying to lose weight, your carbohydrate intake should fall within 100 to 150 grams each day. The sources of carbohydrates should primarily be vegetables and fruit. You can also eat small amounts of healthy starches, such as sweet potatoes and potatoes (with the skin), as well as whole grains, such as brown rice and oats.

Many people wonder if fruits are healthy, as they are sweet and can add back fat to the body. In reality, fruit contains fructose, which is a more complex chemical than sucrose, which is present in sugar. So if your body is exposed to both, it will take more effort for it to digest the former than the latter. In the process, it ends up burning more fat from the body. So don't think eating fruit is bad for you, unless you are eating extremely sweet fruits all throughout the day. However, you might have to exercise precaution if you have high levels of sugar in your body.

Carbohydrates to choose: apples, carrots, oats, quinoa, chickpeas, brown rice, bananas, cauliflower, millet, and kidney beans.

Micronutrients

The body does not need micronutrients in the same amount as macronutrients, but that doesn't mean that they aren't important for the functioning of the body. Micronutrients complement macronutrients by working with them to keep the body moving and are essential to maintaining the right energy levels, cellular function, physical and mental well-being, and metabolism.

The two main micronutrients are vitamins and minerals.

Most people get their micronutrients from plants, which have a large amount of both vitamins and minerals. The amount of micronutrients in a plant depends on the soil that it was grown in. Micronutrients have a wide variety, from vitamin A, B, C, and K to minerals like zinc and magnesium, and all of them are essential for the body.

Chapter Two: Calories

Calories have received a somewhat negative reputation in recent decades, thanks to various fad diets and the tendency to discuss calories as unwanted things. In reality, calories are essential to our survival: if we do not eat enough calories on a daily basis, our bodies will not have the energy required to continue to function, and eventually, our bodies will break down.

All foods are a combination of three building blocks, and these are carbohydrates, proteins, and fats. The calories in each macronutrient are as follows:

- Carbohydrates – 4 calories

- Proteins – 4 calories

- Fats – 9 calories

Sugars, proteins, and fats are each broken down by the body into different compounds, which are then used by the body for different functions. Proteins, fats, and sugars each play an important role in the body, and it is essential to ensure that you are taking in enough of each so that your body has the energy and other resources that it needs to carry out all of its functions.

Calorie Needs

It is difficult to identify exactly how many calories our cells require to function properly, as each person's daily physical activities vary, along with his or her height, weight, age, and gender. To know approximately how many calories you need to consume per day so that you can achieve your weight loss goals, there are three crucial factors that you need to be aware of: Basal Metabolic Rate or BMR, Thermic Effect of Food, and Physical Activity.

These three factors need to be calculated, and by adding up the calculations from these, the result would be the total amount of calories required by your body each day. There are many calorie counters available online, all of which give different results based on the formulas they use. Adding the above three factors is the best and most accurate way to determine the amount of calories needed per day.

Here's a starting point for the number of calories you should be eating if you live a sedentary lifestyle.

For men (to maintain weight):

- Ages 19–30 should eat anywhere from 2,400 to 2,600.

- Ages 31–50 should eat anywhere from 2,200 to 2,400.

- Ages 51 and up should eat anywhere from 2,000 to 2,200.

For women (to maintain weight):

* Recommended: 1,600 to 2,000

Basal Metabolic Rate (BMR) – A person's BMR refers to the amount of energy required for his or her body to function while at rest, that is, for the lungs to continue breathing, the heart to keep pumping, the kidneys to keep functioning, and the body temperature to remain stable. These functions take up approximately 60% to 70% of the calories that are burned during the day. On average, the BMR of men is higher than that of women.

Age is an important factor in the formula because BMR tends to decline by 1% to 2% per decade after you turn 20, largely due to continued loss of fat-free mass in the body. This is, of course, a generalization, and it can differ among individuals depending on exercise, diet, and a person's percentage of body fat.

There are numerous formulas to calculate BMR, and they can be a little complicated. So you can use an online tool to calculate your BMR for you.

Physical Activity – After BMR, this is the second main factor that burns considerable amounts of calories. This includes all that you do with your body, such as walking to work, swimming at the pool, and talking to your friend. The amount of calories that are burned off from physical activity depends on your body weight. The more weight you have, the more calories you burn off as you engage in a particular physical activity. However, if you keep eating as many calories (if not more) as you burn off, you will continue to maintain your current weight (if not increase it).

A great tool to use to calculate how many calories each activity burns is at bitelog.com/exercise-search.htm, but many other online resources can help you to figure out how many calories you are burning.

While many people automatically think of activities like running or going to the gym as the best options for burning calories, there are many other activities that you can choose that will do a great job of burning calories. If you are one of those people, who prefer to disguise exercise in a fun activity; some of these options will work well for you.

Hiking and rock climbing are two excellent examples of fun, outdoor activities that will also help you burn a large number of calories. Depending on the difficulty of the trail and how quickly you are walking, you can burn around 400 calories per hour while hiking, whereas rock climbing can burn from 500 to 700 calories per hour. The difference in calories burned for rock climbing comes from how much you weigh because you are using your own body as the weight in this exercise. On days when the weather is not great, indoor rock climbing is always a great alternative.

If you have some household chores that need to get done and think you don't have time to exercise, think again: those chores are exercise! Vacuuming, laundry, sweeping, and mopping will all burn calories, and using those online resources mentioned earlier can help you figure out just how many calories each chore will burn. If you wash your car, it will burn about 200 calories per hour, and mowing the lawn (using a push mower, not a riding mower!) will burn around

300 calories per hour. Checking items off the "to-do list" and burning calories both make this option a great combination.

Playing sports is perhaps an obvious way to burn calories, but it still should be mentioned because it's a great way to have fun with your friends and still get your exercise in. Football can burn around 500 calories per hour, assuming that you and your friends are somewhat serious about the game, while soccer can burn 600 calories or even more per hour. Even badminton, which is a much lower impact sport, can burn between 250 and 400 calories depending on how much you weigh.

Thermic Effect of Food – This is the last factor that burns the calories that you consume, and it refers to the amount of energy that the body utilizes to digest the food that you have consumed. After all, it does take energy to digest the foods and then break them down into the basic organic compounds that the cells need to function properly.

To determine the number of calories that your body utilizes for this, what you do is multiply the total number of calories consumed within a day by 10%.

24

Chapter Three: Good Fats and Protein

Good Fats

Not all fats are bad for you; eating the right kind of fat will help you lose weight and build lean muscle, but remember that fat contains nine calories per gram, making it more than twice as dense as protein and carbohydrates (each of which has four calories per gram). Eating the right amount of healthy or good fats will help keep you feeling full longer, thus assisting in the weight loss process.

Your body also needs "healthy" fats to manage your mood, achieve top brain function, fight fatigue, and control weight. Your brain, for example, is almost 60% fat – this means that it needs fat to develop and function properly. These healthy fats can also help lower your cholesterol and the risk of heart disease, among other health benefits.

The "unhealthy" fats, on the other hand, can raise your risk of heart disease and increase your cholesterol, as well as cause a variety of other negative health outcomes. This is why it is essential to understand which fats are good and which are bad, as well as to focus on eating the ones that will help your body.

There are four main types of fat found in today's diet of foods developed from plants and animals: monounsaturated, polyunsaturated, trans fats, and saturated fats. Monounsaturated fats and polyunsaturated fats are considered to be the "good" fats, as they provide health benefits. Trans fats are definitively within the "bad" fats category, whereas saturated fats are still somewhat open to debate in the world of nutrition.

Omega-3 fatty acids are one of the most well known types of polyunsaturated fats, and they provide a phenomenal amount of health benefits. These benefits include: preventing and reducing symptoms of ADHD, depression, and bipolar disorder; preventing memory loss and dementia; reducing the risk of stroke, heart disease, and cancer; easing the symptoms of joint pain, arthritis, and inflammatory skin conditions; and supporting a healthy and viable pregnancy.

The best sources for omega-3s are fish, such as salmon, herring, anchovies, oysters, and lake trout. For those who are vegetarian or do not eat fish for other reasons, there are other options: algae, walnuts, Brussels sprouts, spinach, flaxseed, and kale, to name a few.

It is easy to distinguish the good fats from the bad or unhealthy ones. Overall, as indicated above, the "good" fats will be monounsaturated and polyunsaturated fats, which include omega-3s. However, other factors need to be considered when deciding on the specific foods that you will eat and determining whether they are providing good fats or bad fats.

In addition to trans fats, and possibly saturated fats, unhealthy fats are those that have undergone chemical alteration or processing, especially from plant-based fat sources. Meat or dairy fat sources that come from farm-raised animals or mass production are also unhealthy.

Protein

Protein is an essential macronutrient or building block that is known for repairing and creating muscle tissues. It is an essential part of fitness nutrition because it not only helps you lose weight but also promotes lean muscle growth. Now, when you hear the saying "lean protein," it refers to protein sources that have low fat content.

Aside from building lean muscle mass, eating lean protein also makes you feel full for longer periods of time, which in turn will minimize your food consumption and help you lose weight.

In reality, if you are eating the required minimum amount of calories per day, then you are most likely consuming enough protein. However, to build lean muscle mass, it is important to consider your sources of protein to ensure that this nutrient is coming with a well-balanced mixture of other nutritional elements.

Consuming protein helps your body burn more calories than fats or carbohydrates. Approximately 20% to 30% of the calories from proteins go toward the digestion process, while the range is between 5% and 15% for fats and carbohydrates. This is because protein is made up of amino acids, which are held by strong peptide bonds. Your body needs to be able to break down those bonds so that it can use the amino acids to repair tissues and to move oxygen through your bloodstream to form antibodies. To break those bonds, your digestion process has to work overtime, which ultimately results in it drawing more energy.

Remember, though, that just because you are getting more of your calories from protein instead of carbohydrates and fats does not mean that you can eat as many calories as you want. If you eat more calories, you will still gain weight, regardless of whether those calories are coming from protein or other sources.

The best time to eat protein is about 30 to 45 minutes after your workout, regardless of whether you were doing cardio activities or strength training. During that window, your muscles are particularly focused on rebuilding and on repairing the micro-tears that form when you work out. If you give your body protein, that rebuilding and repairing process will work even better, making you less sore the day after and improving your lean muscle mass.

To get the most out of the protein that you are eating, choose a snack that has 12 to 14 grams of protein with a calorie amount of around 40% of what you burned during your workout. So, for example, if you burned 300 calories on the elliptical, choose a snack that contains about 120 calories. Picking a snack that also contains some carbohydrates will help even more with muscle repair and energy replenishment.

The major sources of lean protein are the following: fish, soy, poultry, eggs, mushrooms, beef, beans, peas, lentils, seitan, and dairy. You will notice that there are both vegetarian and non-vegetarian options here, and just because you fall into one of these categories does not mean you cannot attain lean muscles. While meat, poultry, eggs, fish, and dairy do contain all nine amino acids that we get from food – which is why they are often referred to as "complete proteins" – it is very possible to get all of the amino acids from plant-based foods if you eat a balanced variety of such foods. So stop making excuses, and start doing all the right things for your body.

You need to keep in mind that having too much protein isn't a good thing, especially if you aren't working out. In fact, you only need between 40 and 50 grams of protein daily. If you aren't working out, this is a lot of protein and can do more harm than good. So, if you are working out, you need to make sure to get a good amount of protein in your system every day so you can effectively do your workouts. The protein will give you the energy you need to get through all the workouts and will keep you going beyond that.

Chapter Four: Foods to Avoid

Among the things that are proven unhealthy or even devastating in the long term, food is the first that comes to mind. Unhealthy food includes sugary drinks, pizzas, white bread, margarine, vegetable oils, pastries, cookies and cakes, French fries, ice cream, candy bars, processed meat, cheese, artificial sweeteners, and many others.

Sugary Drinks – If we were on a mission to find the unhealthiest product today, we would end up with added sugar. However, it must be emphasized that not all sources of sugar are bad. In the sea of unhealthy products full of sugar, the most important or the unhealthiest are sugary drinks. Many people don't realize that drinks also have calories and, because of that, they fail to understand that drinks can also be bad for health. Sugary drinks include sodas, fruit punches, lemonades, energy drinks, and other drinks with added sugar. Constant consumption of sugary drinks leads to obesity, which can have devastating effects on the human body. Surprisingly, fruit juices are also included in this category. Although they have more nutrients, they also contain very high levels of sugar and calories, which can be very easily neglected by people.

To avoid what was previously mentioned, people must abandon the practice of consuming sugary drinks and search for alternatives, such as water, soda water, tea, and many others. Among the drinks with the most sugar per ounce are the fruit juices, with a range of 4.75 to 7.15 grams of sugar per ounce, followed by regular sodas, energy drinks, iced tea, coffee, and sports drinks.

Pizzas – Pizza is the ultimate favorite food for so many of us. However, only a few of us understand the danger that pizza poses to our health. Similar to sugary drinks, pizza is also one of the reasons for the growing rate of obesity in the world. As regards the number of calories, 100 grams of pizza contain 266 calories, which is for sure a number you don't want to be a part of your daily eating habits. Aside from calories, some pizzas contain 1,620 mg of sodium and 33 grams of fat. One slice of cheese pizza also contains 5 grams of sugar.

However, not all pizzas are marked as unhealthy. To avoid the high intake of calories, fat, sugar, and other unhealthy nutrients, people often choose a vegetable pizza. Vegetable pizza contains vitamins A and C and more fiber in comparison to cheese or meat pizza. Add to this some veggie toppings, such as mushrooms, spinach, tomatoes, or onions, and you will get not only an amazing pizza but also a healthy intake of vitamins and other healthy nutrients.

White Bread – In the majority of cases, white bread is made of wheat, which contains gluten, and because of this, white bread is not good for people who are sensitive to gluten. However, white bread is bad not only for gluten-sensitive people but also for everybody else. White bread is mostly made of refined wheat, the healthy nutrients of which are reduced to a minimum because of the refining process. What you get in the end are pure calories, which can result in high blood pressure for some people. If you want to use bread, it is better to use whole grain bread instead of white bread. Whole grain bread contains a lot more vitamins, minerals, and fiber than white bread. All of this provides you with more energy throughout the day. One slice of white bread has 66 calories, 0.82 grams of fat, 12.65 grams of carbs, and 1.91 grams of protein. Yes, you do get some protein with white bread, but the damage the white bread is causing is much bigger than the benefits of the proteins it contains.

Specialty Coffee Drinks – Fancy coffee drinks with a variety of delicious flavorings are a popular option for many people, but unfortunately, these drinks tend to be extremely high in calories. The problems with these coffee drinks are the same as those with sugary drinks discussed above: empty calories and little, if any, nutritional value. Moreover, we tend to add sugar (or artificial sweeteners) and milk or cream to these drinks, increasing the caloric content even further.

Plain black coffee can help with weight loss because caffeine will boost your metabolism. Adding low fat or part-skim milk is fine, but try to avoid adding sugar or sweeteners.

Processed Meat – Unlike unprocessed meat, processed meat is proven to have negative effects on your health. Several studies around the world indicated that some serious diseases, such as colon cancer, diabetes, and heart disease, could be the result of the consumption of processed meat. If we were to look for a definition of processed meat, it would be that processed meat refers to meat that has been cured, salted, dried, canned, and smoked. In the category of processed meat, we can include hotdogs, sausages, salami, bacon, and ham.

According to some studies, processed meat contains N-nitroso compounds that are proven to be cancer-causing elements. The most important thing about the intake of processed meat is self-control. You must be able to determine the maximum amount of processed meat you are going to eat and decide on what type of processed meat you will be eating because not all types of processed meat are equally unhealthy.

Conclusion

Nutrition is not as simple as just learning about things. You have to apply your knowledge to your everyday routine and make sure that you genuinely change your lifestyle to include things that are better for your health.

Before you make any substantial changes regarding what you eat, you should consult your doctor. This is important just to make sure that you all your nutritional requirements are being met.

More importantly, to attain a healthier lifestyle, you need to motivate yourself to do better. You can keep a diary where you can record all the positive changes in your life or something like a before/after picture. These little things will help push you to cut out all the unhealthy food from your life.

Make sure that you have your friends and family supporting you throughout this process.

Thank you, and remember to share how well these meal planning and organization tips work for you. You can do that by writing a review in your Amazon account under Your Orders.

Thank you,

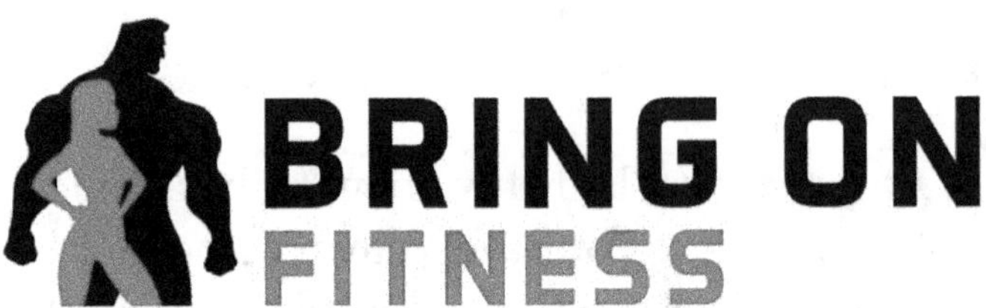

Resources

http://www.eatright.org/resources/food/nutrition

https://www.bornfitness.com/fix-your-diet-understanding-proteins-carbs-and-fats/

https://www.medicalnewstoday.com/articles/263028.php

https://www.nhs.uk/Livewell/loseweight/Pages/understanding-calories.aspx

Book 2
Meal Planning

A Beginners Guide to Meal Planning

By

Bring On Fitness

About Bring On Fitness

Our passion for fitness gave life to **Bring On Fitness**. We started with the goal of helping as many people as we can. To educate, motivate and to help change peoples lives for the better. Bring On Fitness is not only for the fitness enthusiasts, but also for the beginner. We strongly believe nothing is more important than learning the basics and creating a strong foundation in both nutrition - through meal planning, and in exercise - by following a specific plan. This is just as important for the beginner, as it is for the experienced athlete.

We set high standards for ourselves, the information we share, and the products we carry. Our goal is to provide you with exceptional products that suit your needs and the knowledge and motivation to help you work towards and achieve your health and fitness goals.

Check us out at www.bringonfitness.com

"Our Mission is to have a positive impact in changing peoples lives. We will deliver the best possible fitness and nutrition solutions that will empower people to achieve their health and fitness goals."

Table of Contents

Introduction

Meal planning is one of the best ways to maintain a budget, your weight, and overall health. Meal planning allows you to set out your meals on a daily, weekly, or monthly basis. It helps you determine your shopping list and avoid extraneous purchases while you are in a store.

Meal planning begins with recipes, with foods that you know you are going to want to eat, which is why you ultimately save time, maintain your budget, and can control your weight. You are going to choose meals that are healthy and that you could work in the time frame you have to prepare the meals, which will ensure you are not eating out as often.

You can choose any time to plan meals, organize your shopping list, and prep on a daily, weekly, or monthly basis. With meal planning, you and will start to eat healthy, home-cooked meals. After a month of following the meal planning techniques, you are going to see how cost effective it is and why more people are trying to change their habits and routines.

It does not matter where you are; whether you are at home, using a few spare minutes at work or on public transportation, you can plan your meals on the way to work, at home or at work.

You are going to learn how to use cookbooks, magazines, online sites, software, and grocery lists to plan your meals. You are also going to discover why storage containers and crockpots are necessary for meal planning and meal organization.

Stop letting your cravings and hunger rule you as you leave work. Do not let pizza, fast food, or other restaurants tempt you. With proper meal planning techniques and better meal organization, you can have a hot, home-cooked meal as soon as you arrive home.

Chapter 1: Materials to Plan and Organize

Planning takes a little preparation and organization. It is all rolled into the new routine you are going to undertake for healthier meals. Getting started with planning is made easier when you have the right materials for the type of person you are.

For example, people from an older generation are going to grab a paper and pencil to make out his grocery list. What about you? Are you at an age where you get your computer or phone to check an item in a meal planning program, or do you take to your Amazon Dot, Google Home, or Apple equivalent and have your device create a shopping list that is tied to your phone?

Your first step is to decide whether you want to use tech or not for your shopping list. The wonderful thing about technology is you can add anything to your phone, whether you are home, at work, or on the go, thus saving yourself from forgetting what you just thought of to add to the list.

You can also use pre-made shopping lists. These nutrition lists tell you what you should be buying to have nutritious meals every time. For example, they are broken down into protein, carbohydrates, fats, and other health categories. You are supposed to make sure you are buying the food on each section of the list that is healthiest for you. These lists are available through software and online nutrition programs. You can download the sheet and print it, create your own, or merely establish a shopping list of items you like and print it each time you go to the store.

Delving into Organization

The shopping list is the natural part. There are still plenty of things you need to do to get organized so that you can plan your meals.

1. Purchase a set of storage containers. You want different sizes and preferably a few pieces in that set that allow you to freeze food without it getting freezer burned.

2. Buy meal containers. There are salad containers, where you can put your lettuce, meat, cheese, and other cold items in the bottom, and place things like croutons and salad dressing on top, helping to keep everything fresh. Bento boxes are available around the world, even in the U.S. Bento boxes are meal storage containers designed by the Japanese to have their rice, meat, and vegetables in their "lunch" box.

3. Have a crockpot or three. Crockpots are a fantastic way to have a home-cooked meal hot when you arrive home. We have come a long way with crockpots, making them Wi-Fi and Bluetooth connected. Moreover, they have timers so that you can set it on high or low, then after a specific time, change the setting from high to low and low to warm. It provides the perfect meal. Added to that, Crockpot has a version with three pots in one. You have a six-quart, four-quart, and three-quart pot. The three-quart pot is split into two, so you can make two different dishes.

Finding Meals to Plan

Obtaining the materials, such as how you will generate your shopping list and what items you will use for the preparation portion of your meal planning, naturally leads into the last piece of organization, which is how to locate the meals you intend on planning and executing.

- Use cookbooks you already have.

- Find favored recipes in magazines you have.

- Look through new magazines.

- Set online alerts at recipe sites.

We get tired of eating the same things. We want to do something different, but then we begin to think about how much time it will take to accomplish these meals. Part of meal planning and organization is ensuring that you can cut down the time it takes for you to prepare the meal on busy days.

Recipes are not going to be offered here, but there are some suggestions on how you can minimize your cooking time.

Do you use every recipe in a cookbook that you own? Did you buy a book for one or two recipes? Perhaps, there was a magazine you kept because it had something you wanted to try. You can eliminate the clutter in your kitchen and save only the recipes you use.

Whether you tear the recipes out of the magazine or write it out on a recipe card, you can become more organized in your meal planning by making the recipes handier. Quite a few libraries carry magazines, including food magazines, so you do not have to buy the periodical to access new recipes. You can borrow the journal, write down the information, and return it.

Many of the websites offering recipes provide current updates each day. They might send you a reminder for the recipe of the day, outlining a little of the meal to entice you to log in and download the recipe. You have plenty of options when it comes to finding new ways to make food.

You can even search for five-ingredient recipes online and in select books that are meant to minimize the food you have to prep for a decent meal.

Chapter 2: Daily, Weekly, or Monthly Prep

Most of us avoid cooking because of the work it takes to make a meal. In an hour or thirty minutes, you might be done with cooking the meal, but you eat it in fifteen minutes. All the work seems silly when you enjoy it quickly and move on to the next portion of your day.

However, you can help eliminate these feelings that prevent you from cooking. Later, you will learn how to accept the cleanup portion that also makes you hesitate to cook every meal.

For now, let's focus on the options for meal prep. Typically, you consider meal prep to be what you do right before you start cooking. This is the part where you wash the vegetables, slice the meat, and take out the various sauces, spices, and herbs you are going to use.

You have three options for how you want to tackle the preparation of food:

1. Daily

2. Weekly

3. Monthly

Meal planning is about organizing your life better, which means prepping food promptly.

Daily Prep

Daily preparation is about making sure you have three meals planned, prepped, and ready for you. Daily preparation is best done at night or first thing in the morning. Most people are too busy in the morning, trying to get kids and spouses up and fed before going to work. You may be just as busy at night with seeing to it that the kids do their homework, are fed, and get to bed on time. After they go to bed, you want to relax and watch TV or read.

For the person who watches a lot of television, you can combine your meal prep with TV. With streaming services, through multiple devices like tablets and affordable TVs, you can watch your show while cutting vegetables for the next day.

Daily preparation is advantageous if you live near farmer's markets year-round or have access to fresh produce stores. You can shop daily and keep all the food fresh. For example, you can stop at the store before you go home after work, get fresh items, and prep them for the next day.

It is during this preparation period that you are going to use your storage containers. You will have various-sized containers, purchased as part of your new meal planning strategy that you can use for the different ingredients you will need.

You do not have to go crazy and label each one or use a different one for each ingredient. For example, a recipe may tell you to combine white vinegar with soy sauce, pepper, orange juice, and honey. You could combine all those ingredients into one container. You could also put the meat in it to soak longer than the thirty minutes. The point is that with specific recipes and ingredients, you can combine items. If you make a stir-fry, you will mix water chestnuts and carrots in one container because they require the same amount of cook time, but have the bamboo shoots and broccoli in a separate container.

If you are a hyper-organized person, you might want to use a label maker to mark everything. If you are going to use specific vegetables for all three meals, you may combine them in one container and have separate bins for each vegetable and fruit. It all depends on the recipe, but the main point is for you to organize your ingredients based on what you are going to use, considering the amounts and what is most comfortable when it comes time to prepare the meal.

The next day, you grab the stacked containers that you need, warm the pan, oven, or pot, and begin making your meal.

Weekly Prep

Preparing meals on a weekly basis can be more natural, just as it is harder because of habits you may have. At the beginning of the week, you may have particular cravings but find later in the week that you are not as keen on a specific meal. However, you are stuck with what you have prepared; therefore, you will either make something among the meals you prepped or eat out.

On the other hand, when you have meals planned and ready to make, you do not have to worry about going home, throwing it in a pot or pan, and having a meal in a few minutes. It can make things easier when you know you do not have time at night or during the day to prep the next days' meals.

Weekly preparation of meals is going to take a lot of energy and at least half a day, if not the entire day, to get everything ready.

You will start by choosing the recipes, getting the ingredients you need, and prepping the meal as far as possible. Typically, this is about cutting vegetables, portioning out the seasonings, spices, and herbs you are going to use, and ensuring that you just have to grab each container as needed when you start cooking.

Your fridge, as well as the cabinet where you have decided to put the dry or non-refrigerator ingredients, will be organized by meal. You do not want a stack on your counter, so you are going to need space for the items that you do not need to put in the fridge.

For the weekly prep, it is better to have labels to avoid grabbing the wrong containers. It is helpful because you may have specific portions that you do not want to mix up. As an example, you may need a meal for two one night and a meal for four the next night, which means portions should be labeled accordingly.

Weekly prep is excellent when you do not have farmer's markets on a daily basis or access to the freshest produce. Mountain towns, for example, tend to have your typical grocery store, so going more than once a week is not going to ensure the items are any fresher. There may also be a summer farmer's market, but then nothing in the winter months. It does not make sense in some places to shop each day at the store; thus, going to a fresh produce and meat market on a weekly basis may fit better with what you have around you for shopping.

Monthly Prep

Like weekly prep, you need to carve out a day each month to prepare all the food you want to make during the month. You can decide to have a new meal each day or repeat your menu. Monthly preparation makes the most sense when you are on a strict budget. When you know you cannot afford steak each week, but only once a month, and will be eating mostly chicken and hamburger meals, you can prepare ingredients on a monthly basis.

You have several options to be hyper-organized, such as freezing vegetables, fruits, and cut meats. It is not the healthiest option when you have to buy in bulk and freeze things, but it is also not as bad as continuing to eat out at the cheapest fast food restaurants.

Monthly organization for meals can include accessing better ways to purchase items based on your meal planning. Warehouse stores are good for buying cheap meat, chicken, and bulk items to help you freeze and store the food you are going to eat for the month.

Moreover, depending on where you live, you might consider the value of buying fresh meat from a local farmer. In the west and mid-west, it is common to find local farmers who sell cow meat by the quarter, half, or full. For a better cost than most stores, you can have plenty of hamburger, roasts, and steaks. One person purchased a quarter of a cow, which was 108 pounds of meat, for $6.00 per pound. The order included four T-bone steaks, 23 pounds of hamburger, and much more. Imagine a T-bone steak for $6.00 per pound. It provides a way for you to get a variety. Of course, you may need to know someone or live in an area where this is customary practice.

Overall, there are options to prepare your meals on a daily, weekly, or monthly basis, where you are eating healthier meals based on the planning you have done and what you are most likely to eat throughout the year.

Last Tips for Prepping Meals

Most of the time, meal prep is about organizing the ingredients you purchase based on the meals you plan, but not cooking anything. You do have another option. You can choose quite a few recipes that allow you to cook most of the meal and leave only a little cooking for the day you are going to eat. For example, baked eggs, like an egg casserole, can be cooked the evening before and reheated throughout the week in a portion that fits your needs.

You can also bake several things like muffins, overnight French toast, and more grain-based foods to eat for breakfast throughout the week. Making muffins and freezing them is one way to have fresh fruit in a muffin when you are in the mood instead of each day.

These are the points you need to think about as you plan the meals you enjoy and buy your ingredients.

Chapter 3: Daily or Weekly Cooking

Like the preparation of ingredients, you have the option of when you are going to cook. In the previous section, you were left with ideas of potential meal options that you could cook on a weekly or monthly basis and store. Here are some additional tips based on the daily or weekly preparation you may wish to do for your meals.

Daily Tips

- To stay organized, you will need to use meal containers.

- You can prep the menu items and cook them the day you want to eat the meal, or you can cook everything the day before and reheat it.

- Crockpots allow you to cook your dinner while you are at work and come home to a warm meal.

- Overnight recipes or things like egg meals are easy to prepare the night before and reheat right before you run out the door.

- You can also cook lunches the night before, so you have a hot meal at work by reheating it.

- Smoothies are also a way to get your health benefits with minimal fuss. Smoothies can be frozen, already blended, and thawed, with a quick turn in the blender before you run out the door.

Weekly Tips

Cooking on a weekly basis is more about taking one day that you cook several meals, store them in meal containers, and grab them from the freezer on your way out the door. You can do this with a variety of options, although some recipes work better. Just think about all the frozen meals you find in the grocery store, and consider which recipes you like the most but know you can make fresher and healthier.

Lasagna, spaghetti pie, omelet style-eggs, bacon, sausage, Asian dishes, Salisbury steak, chicken fried steak, chicken tenders, and much more can be on your weekly menu and all cooked and frozen.

The ideas are limitless. However, the point is not to focus on recipes but to ensure you are planning meals you are going to eat.

What you should desire is to find things you love to eat and figure out a way you can be comfortable with preparing everything and cooking them on a weekly basis versus daily.

Have you considered making fresh pasta, cooking it, and then freezing it? You could go with the right Kitchen Aid contraptions, such as a ravioli pasta maker. Just freeze the ravioli when you are done, and cook them as needed, or cook them with the sauce added and then freeze the entire meal.

By using meal containers that have each portion of the meal sectioned, you can heat it up or eat it when you are ready.

The benefit of weekly cooking is that you can come home and eat right away versus having to grab all the ingredients and cooking before you can eat.

Chapter 4: Dieting and Meal Planning

By now, you understand that meal planning is all about deciding what you can do based on your time and willingness. Some people are more willing to come home and prepare their meals each night, whereas others have a weekday or weekend they can cook all their meals and save time throughout the week.

However, can you continue to follow a regimented diet if you are planning your meals? It is even easier for you to stay on a diet when you use meal planning. Think about some of the diets you have started but stopped because of the preparation of the meals or the lack of time.

Any diet that exists can conform to meal planning because setting up your meals is about buying the ingredients and organizing your life so that you can save time when you lack it to give to your diet.

You also have a better hand on the portion control required for dieting. For example, Weight Watchers was all about calorie counting in the past, where you could add points up based on the types of food you were eating for the day. Sometimes, you could have dessert because you watched your points, but the time it took to count your menu items was aggravating.

What if you use meal planning to create recipes that work for your diet, where you already have the correct portions and food items, and you no longer have to think about what you are doing on a daily basis?

The benefit of meal planning is precisely the answer to the question. Whether you plan, prep, and cook all in one day or on a daily basis, you can weigh your food portions, cut the meats to the right sizes, and ensure you are always eating a well-balanced meal.

Imagine how healthy you can feel when you no longer give into your cravings or want dessert because you did not eat enough food during the day.

How does this work? Well, let's take a look at the way you can use meal planning for dieting.

1. Meal planning works on any diet.

2. Planning out the meals you will eat during the day or throughout the week helps you stick to your diet.

3. Prepping the ingredients gives you healthy choices based on your mood or cravings.

4. Cooking also prevents you from suddenly eating out because you know there is a meal ready to reheat at home.

Watching your Habits

For meal planning to work in combination with a diet, you need to understand the habits you have and how you can modify them. For men, it is a little easier to plan meals without giving in to cravings because hormones are not going to interfere with you each month.

As a woman, there are times that chocolate, ice cream, and all the junk food in the world call out, begging you to eat these foods. However, if you know your habits, you can combat these issues.

- When do you feel the need for junk food?

- When do you find yourself buying things that are not as healthy?

- What meals have you eaten often?

- What ingredients do you buy and tend to waste?

- Why do you avoid cooking?

- How much sleep do you get at night?

- Are you stressed or worried?

By answering the above questions, you can begin to track your habits and learn from them. Meal planning is as much a time concept as it is correcting your overall habits.

For example, are you thinking everything written in previous sections and this diet chapter sounds excellent, but you do not have the time or energy? What if you learn that energy and time can be found, if you begin to have a healthier lifestyle, which starts with proper meal planning?

It is all about falling into a new cycle. What will you do the next time you have a craving for something, but did not plan it as part of your daily or weekly meal? Will you succumb to your desire, or will you stand firm by using your mind to talk your psyche out of the desire?

Eating healthier because you are planning your meals is definitely about overcoming your mind. It is also about starting the trek to healthier eating, so you have more energy, are more robust, and stop craving the junk. Did you know that eating more fruit satisfies your body as regards sugar? At first, you might want ice cream and other sugar-laden food, but once you start eating fruit in place of desserts and for mid-day snacks, your body begins to desire the fruit instead of the ice cream.

Overcoming the cravings by planning meals is possible.

The one thing you cannot do is quit your habits cold turkey, as this sets you up for failure.

Planning Meals with Slow Changes

You can start your meal planning concept slowly, whether you are going to diet or not.

1. Begin planning three meals for one day a week.

2. Choose a day you have off.

3. Look at what you have in your home. What recipes can you use based on the foods you already have?

4. Go shopping if your fridge and cabinets are empty.

5. Buy only what you need for the day.

6. Return from the store and prep as much as you want. If it is just vegetables and fruits that you wash, cut, and store, that is fine. You can go all the way by cutting the

meat and combining the spices and sauces or merely go half way.

7. When mealtime comes, cook.

8. Clean up immediately and during the meal.

Clean up is one of the most challenging aspects of prepping the meals. Planning is easy on paper, but the execution is the tough part. It is suggested that you take your time by adding a day at a time to your meal planning, prep, and organizing because you can see how enjoyable it is to come home to cooked meals or at least prepped meals.

You also give your body a chance to become healthier. You work on your body to trick it into liking the healthy meals versus the ones that end with dessert or junk food.

Eventually, you gain energy enough to enjoy the preparation portion of the organization. You will sleep better because your body is happier from eating correctly.

If you are stressed or worried, meal planning is not going to help with that; however, you should find a way to alleviate your situation. Anyone who is depressed or feeling too much worry will have a harder time changing habits, but it is possible. Just remember, take things one step at a time; this leads to a healthier you, and sometimes, you may fall back into old patterns, but get back up. Try again, and you will succeed.

Conclusion

Meal planning offers you several options for a healthier life, whether or not you decide to diet during your change to a better lifestyle.

It is going to take time to change the habits you have had for the last several years, but stick to meal planning, and you will enjoy a healthier way of eating.

Start your planning today, as soon as you finish reading this. Your task is to look at what you have in your kitchen, and decide what you can make for the next meal. Find a recipe, or go with one you love. Outline it, cut the ingredients, and store them. Cook them when you are ready to eat.

Next, when you revisit a shop for whatever you need regarding meal planning, buy all new storage and meal containers. Starting out with new things, with assorted sizes and designs, gives you an emotional fist pump. You will be excited about using those new containers and want to go home to start immediately. It may sound silly, but it does work.

Find what works for you

The last tip that can be offered in summation is for you to remember the golden rule—you can always modify your plan. Toss what does not work, and keep what does. After a week of meal planning, if something does not work, change, and find out what does. For example, if you tried the daily planning and prep, try the weekly concept. You might find a combination of weekly and daily planning works best based on your time constraints.

Thank you, and remember to share how well these meal planning and organization tips work for you. You can do that by writing a review in your Amazon account under Your Orders.

Thank you,

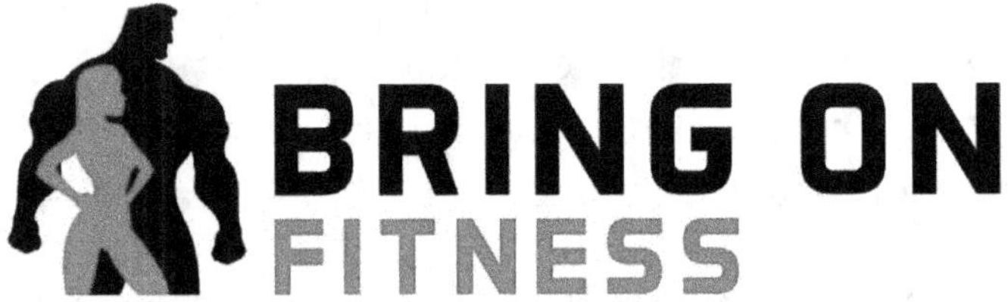

Book 3
Weight Loss

20 Reasons Why You Are Not Losing Weight

By

Bring on Fitness

About Bring On Fitness

Our passion for fitness gave life to **Bring On Fitness**. We started with the goal of helping as many people as we can. To educate, motivate and to help change peoples lives for the better. Bring On Fitness is not only for the fitness enthusiasts, but also for the beginner. We strongly believe nothing is more important than learning the basics and creating a strong foundation in both nutrition - through meal planning, and in exercise - by following a specific plan. This is just as important for the beginner, as it is for the experienced athlete.

We set high standards for ourselves, the information we share, and the products we carry. Our goal is to provide you with exceptional products that suit your needs and the knowledge and motivation to help you work towards and achieve your health and fitness goals.

Check us out at www.bringonfitness.com

"Our Mission is to have a positive impact in changing peoples lives. We will deliver the best possible fitness and nutrition solutions that will empower people to achieve their health and fitness goals."

Table of Contents

Introduction

You cannot stand in line at the supermarket or flip through television channels without seeing people celebrated for their thin, attractive bodies. Some people have worked hard to maintain their physique, while others rely on Photoshop and other techniques to make them appear thinner.

Regardless, it puts a lot of pressure on people to lose weight. This can be seen in crazes over weight loss fads, including workout plans, diets, and miracle supplements that are intended to help us lose weight quickly. There is such an obsession with looking great that there is a huge market for the weight loss industry and plenty of ways for companies to capitalize on the desires of others. In America alone, nearly $60 billion is spent on weight loss methods, including low-calorie foods, bariatric surgery, diet pills, health club memberships, and much more.

The downside of all this money spent is that it is not always effective. In fact, many people who lose weight fail to keep it off. Others try to lose weight and plateau, hitting a standstill before they come close to their weight loss goal. So when it seems like you have tried everything, what do you do?

The truth of the matter is that there are many reasons you may not be losing the weight that you want. Some have to do with your diet, while others have to do with the methods you are using to meet your weight loss goals. The good news is that by learning more about your body and the science behind how it works, you can both achieve and maintain your weight loss.

When it comes to weight loss, there is no such thing as starting tomorrow. Start right now by reading through the pages of this book. By the end, you will have some insight into the reasons why you are having trouble losing weight.

Mistake #1: Your Training Regime is Predictable

One common message for people trying to lose weight is that they should move around more. Even doing small things like walking around more at work, parking further away from the entrance of places of business, and taking the stairs instead of the elevator has been proven to help people increase the number of calories they are burning, thus causing weight loss. However, more recent studies show that there is a maximum point for calorie expenditure. This means that, at some point, even with intense exercise, your body stops burning calories. This means that you could be doing extra work for nothing.

According to the NYU Langone Medical Center Medical Weight Management Program director, Holly Lofton, it is quite common for people who pair extreme workouts with the same dietary habits to plateau with weight loss. It may work at first, especially for those who live a more sedentary lifestyle, but eventually, weight loss comes to a halt.

One thing that you can do to combat this problem is to switch up your workout routine. If you rely on biking or walking to lose weight, try swimming or yoga instead. You can also learn more about your body by finding out at what point you plateau. Each body reacts differently to exercise. For example, someone with a higher body fat percentage is more likely to burn more calories before plateauing than someone with a lower body fat percentage. Factors like muscle mass, genetic markers, metabolism, and hormone levels can also affect how many calories you can burn before reaching that plateau.

Mistake #2: Your Body Cannot Put More Calories Out without Storing Some

Even though evolution has changed the human body in many ways, many of our primitive instincts and patterns still exist. One of these primitive instincts is to survive by ensuring the body has enough calories to perform its regular functions. Associate Professor of Anthropology Herman Pontzer worked with his associates on a study that examined the way the body uses a system of checks and balances to ensure survival when it comes to burning calories.

The study examined people with sedentary lifestyles compared to hunter-gatherer populations in Tanzania. The conclusion was that even though the Tanzanian hunter-gatherers are incredibly active, with the men walking 10 miles per day and the women walking 6 miles, they do not expend more calories than a more sedentary person.

This phenomenon can be explained by dividing calories into two categories—resting calories and activity calories. The resting calories are those that the body stores to ensure that it is functioning in the way it is supposed to. This is necessary to fight against inflammation, keep the immune system healthy, and ensure the body is receiving and responding to signals from the brain. These resting calories are necessary for health.

Outside of the resting calories are the activity calories, which are those that are freed up so they can be burned during physical activity. Once you run out of the activity calories, your body will burn rest calories—but only at a very slow rate. This is a primitive function that ensures health. After all, it does no good to lose weight if your immune system is not functioning properly and you get sick.

Mistake #3: You Are Stressed Out

For a long time, the latest dieting trends were all you heard about for weight loss. Things like restricted-calorie eating, the cabbage soup diet, and other trends could produce results—but only to an extent. Plus, the statistics do not lie. The majority of people who can lose weight with a diet end up gaining that weight back (and often, more weight than they started with) within five years. This is proven by several studies, including one in 2002 that analyzed 231 million dieting Europeans—only 1% were able to attain permanent weight loss following their diet.

One of the reasons that dieting is next to impossible (and ineffective) is because of the stress it causes. Stress is the enemy of dieting for two reasons. First, it increases the body's production of the hormone cortisol. Cortisol is known for causing the body to store fat poorly, especially around the abdominal area.

Additionally, stress is more likely to cause binge eating. This can make you sit down and eat more calories than your body needs—and then store it, as a result. This is incredibly detrimental to weight loss efforts. In this case, it would seem that making lifestyle changes, rather than sticking to a diet, would be a better option for losing weight.

Mistake #4: Metabolic Suppression

One of the most popular shows for weight loss miracles is "The Biggest Loser"—a competition in which the contestants' goal is to lose weight. On average, the contestants lose 129 pounds each. Unfortunately, a study done six years later found that the participants had gained back an average of 70% of the weight they had lost. Additionally, they were burning fewer calories than the average person of their weight and size—about 500 calories less, to be exact.

This study mirrors similar studies that have examined the weight regulation in the mind. This is known as a set point. Basically, each person has a set point for their weight, which their body tries to maintain. When you drop below your body's set point, the mind starts to fight back against dieting.

The brain fights back in a few ways. First, it reduces the number of calories burned during physical activity compared to the calories burned for the average person. This is known as metabolic suppression because the brain is suppressing how quickly the metabolism works. Second, it affects the way you eat. Not only does it produce hunger hormones to encourage you to eat more, it lights up the pleasure center in your brain, such that eating becomes more rewarding.

Mistake #5: You Are Depriving Yourself

Studies done with rats show how food deprivation affects the mind. One study restricted the amount of food that rats were allowed to eat for five days and then gave them unlimited Oreos for two days. This was done for several weeks. Then, a stressor was introduced to the rats with the restricted diet and a control group. The study showed that the rats who were dieting ate twice as many Oreos following exposure to the stressor when compared with the control group. Then, it was noted that even when a single bite of Oreo was eaten, the rats would binge on regular food when it was available.

One of the reasons why diets do not work is because a diet encourages the deprivation mindset. When the body and mind are deprived, whether through calorie restriction or drastic diet changes, it changes the way that neurotransmitters like dopamine work in the brain. It makes eating more pleasurable and causes you to seek out unhealthy foods as a result, to experience this reward.

The same study has also shown that once the dieting period was over, binge eating was still a problem. This may explain why, following a successful diet, people are still likely to gain the weight back. Instead of depriving yourself, consider having a cheat meal. Do not make it a whole day where you binge eat, but know that it is okay to give into your cravings on occasion.

Mistake #6: You Are Eating Too Much

Often, people eat not because they are hungry, but because external cues are telling them that they need the food. The food marketing industry is partly to blame for this, particularly the problem of overeating. It is harder to resist something when you are getting a deal. For example, why get a half-size sub when you can get a full one for just a dollar or two more? When it is only a dollar to supersize a meal and get more food (and more calories), it just seems to make sense to get the larger amount of food. Food selling techniques have also become extreme—with companies even using sexuality to sell things like burgers.

Another problem is falling into negative habits with your food. Imagine that a couple of nights out of the week, you eat a snack and watch television right before bed. This is a poor choice simply because you are eating calories right before you go into a restful state for the night. However, if done regularly, you may find yourself craving snacks just because you are sitting down in front of the television. This leads to eating even when you are not hungry.

The key to overcoming this is learning to eat when you are actually hungry, rather than whenever the thought crosses your mind. Pay attention to physical body cues that indicate you are hungry, like a growling stomach or fatigue that indicates a need to refuel. Then, eat at a slow enough pace that you can register when you start to feel full—and stop eating.

Mistake #7: You Have Trouble Detecting Hunger/Fullness Cues

Many people who have trouble overeating struggle with understanding their own bodies. They may have been used to eating whatever they want whenever they feel like it for so long that they cannot even tell when they are hungry or full. This is a problem because it often leads to eating more food than you need to consume. These extra calories translate to stored fat.

One of the best ways to learn to listen to your body is to start eating in an area that is free of distractions. If this does not work, there may be emotional reasons or an underlying problem that drives you to eat. Discovering this can help you find the root of your problematic relationship with food.

Another technique that you can use is putting smaller portions on your plate. Given that your desire to avoid waste sometimes overwhelms feelings of fullness, making you feel like you must clean your plate, it is better to eat smaller portions.

When you cannot detect the cues at all, the best answer may be eating on a set schedule. Eat a small snack two to three times per day, and eat a meal three times daily. Ideally, you should speak with a nutritionist about the ideal calorie range for someone of your weight who wants to lose weight. Then, fit your meals into this calorie range.

Mistake #8: You Aren't Slowing Down to Eat

Did you know that your body is satisfied with food long before your mind is? While eating nourishes your physical body, it has effects on the mind as well. One of the biggest mistakes that people make is trying to eat their food quickly. This is problematic because it takes time for the food to pass from mouth to stomach and even longer for the brain to register that the body is full.

To overcome this problem, you must start slowing down when you eat. Fully chew each bite, and take a few breaths before going for another one. Pay attention to how your stomach feels as you eat. Once you have fulfilled your needs, you will notice that you are not enjoying the food as much. You may also feel pressure in your stomach. If you overeat, it can cause discomfort, pain, or queasiness. Overeating can also affect your body later on, as it slows down to process your full stomach.

Ideally, by slowly and thoughtfully chewing each bite, you will learn to stop eating when you are full. Many people eat more than their bodies need, and this can make it nearly impossible to lose weight—even when making healthier food choices.

Mistake #9: Your Hunger Cues Are Being Confused with Something Else

Hunger cues are not the only thing that drives you to eat. There are several other triggers that people experience, which can be confused as a signal from the body that you are hungry. These include:

- Mind Hunger – If you develop excessive eating habits, like eating a certain amount of food simply because it is "time" to eat, it can cause you to think you are hungry when you are not.

- Teeth Hunger – Sometimes, the urge to have a cigarette or chew on something comes to you in times of frustration. You are not hungry, but you have an oral fixation that needs to be satisfied. Try chewing a piece of gum instead.

- Mouth Hunger – The smell or sight of food has the potential to make your mouth water and feel hungry, which can bring about cravings unrelated to hunger.

- Emotional Hunger – Food can be pleasurable and even comforting. This is what causes emotional eating in some cases, which is often a result of filling a void by using food or using it to push your feelings down.

- Fatigue – If you are overly tired, lack of food may not be to blame. It can also result from not getting enough sleep or working too hard.

- Thirst – Being thirsty can cause you to feel hungry, often because of the sluggishness that results from dehydration. Try drinking a glass of water when you think you are hungry before you try eating.

Mistake #10: You Are Only Focusing on the Numbers

Often, people who are trying to lose weight are aiming to see a certain number on the scale. The problem is that weight loss does not always result in lower numbers, especially for people who are building muscle tone through exercise during their efforts. This happens because muscle weighs more than fat, so gains in muscle can actually appear as if you are increasing in weight instead of losing it.

There are also other factors that affect weight loss. These include things like water weight, how quickly the foods you are eating are digested, and your bowel movements. If you want a more accurate measurement, consider using how you look and how clothes fit as indicators that you are moving in the right direction.

It is important to remember that weight loss is not so much about hitting a certain number as it is about becoming healthier and improving your fat-to-muscle ratio. Do not focus on the numbers—focus on the results.

Mistake #11: You're Making Efforts, but You Are Not Tracking Them

Many people consume more calories each day than they think—even hundreds more. It is true that making small changes to your diet and lifestyle, such as moving around more and making healthier eating choices, can help with weight loss efforts. If you are not tracking what is happening, however, you may not be doing enough.

In today's age of technology, it is easier than ever to track your calories and activity. There are countless apps and devices designed to help make losing weight significantly easier. Some devices may track calories burned or how far you walk, while others measure sleep patterns and heart rate, too. Even calorie counting apps can be sophisticated, letting you scan bar codes of the foods you eat or input food items to calculate your total caloric intake.

The apps and devices that you choose to work with are ultimately up to you. Keep in mind, however, that by knowing what is working and what isn't, you can drastically improve your efforts.

Mistake #12: You Think That Healthy Foods Have No Calories

When you are trying to lose weight for better health, keep in mind that it is not always the numbers that matter. For your body's metabolism to stay at a healthy rate and for you to diet without feeling hungry, you should seek foods that are wholesome in nature.

Did you know that many diet foods contain processed ingredients that are not-so-healthy for your body? They may be low in calories, but they are also low in nutrition. For example, diet sodas are a popular choice for people looking for a low-calorie soda alternative. However, diet soda has actually been seen to increase people's weight in a few studies, although science is still out on the reasoning behind this.

Instead of seeking out these foods, opt for more wholesome foods. Eat a diet rich in protein, whole grains, and fruits and vegetables. When you are making food choices, do not count calories—make your calories count.

Mistake #13: You Are Not Eating Enough Protein

One of the most important foods for a person who is trying to lose weight is protein. Protein has numerous benefits for people trying to lose weight. One of the first things to note is that when you pay attention to your body cues and eat when you are hungry, protein can stave off hunger. This is because the body digests it slower, so it stays in your stomach longer. Protein consumption also boosts metabolism. Finally, the way that protein affects the brain can also increase weight loss.

High levels of protein can alter the hormones produced by the area of the brain known as the hypothalamus. It is the hypothalamus that helps regulate weight. When you consume higher amounts of protein and reduce fat and carbs, it reduces the production of the hunger hormone and increases the production of satiety hormones that tell your body it is full. This means you may eat fewer calories. For most diets, it is recommended that around 30% of your daily caloric intake should come from protein.

The quality of the protein you are eating can also affect how quickly you are losing weight. Consider lean meats for protein, such as fish, chicken, and hamburger with a lower fat content. Whole grains and beans are other good, wholesome sources of protein.

Mistake #14: You're Skipping Out on the Weights

Many people know the importance of trying to be more active when trying to lose weight, but did you know that regular muscle workouts are an important part of losing and maintaining weight loss? The body is not always picky about what it is burning. If you are not using your muscles regularly, you may find that your dieting regimen is causing you to lose muscle mass in addition to fat. This is because the body will burn this up to make up the reduction in calories, too, especially if you are not working out.

You also will find that you look better once you have lost weight if you continue to tone your muscles. It can help reduce the amount of extra skin that is left behind once you lose weight. Additionally, lifting weights can help keep your metabolism working how it is supposed to, preventing the slow down that can bring your weight loss efforts to a screeching halt.

You do not have to strain yourself to lift weights. Start with a few repetitions of a low weight, even if it is just 10 or 15 pounds. As you increase the weight you are lifting, you will burn more calories and improve the way you look.

Mistake #15: You Are Doing Too Much Low-Intensity Cardio Training

When you are trying to lose weight and get healthier, cardiovascular workouts can speed up your progress. Some workouts, such as jogging and running, have received bad publicity in the last few years because of their impact on joint health, but there are plenty of alternatives that can get your heart pumping fast. This includes swimming, jumping on a trampoline, and using an elliptical machine.

In the past few years, one type of exercise that has received a lot of hype for burning fat is high-intensity interval training or HIIT. During this type of exercise, you keep a steady pace and then you work to increase your heart rate for a set period of time. Then, you take another small break, but keep moving. For example, you would jog for five minutes and then run for two, followed by another period of jogging.

In general, cardiovascular exercise is a critical part of weight loss. It helps burn belly fat, which can be stubborn to get rid of. It also offers numeral health benefits, including reducing your risk of heart disease and eliminating visceral fat, which builds up around the organs.

Mistake #16: You Are Not Sleeping Enough

Studies show that individuals with poor sleeping habits are more likely to be obese. These statistics show a 55% greater risk for adults and an 89% greater risk for children. A study conducted by the University of Chicago uncovered the reason behind this correlation—"metabolic grogginess."

When you do not get enough sleep, the fat cells in your body feel the deprivation. The result is difficulty using insulin, which can lead to insulin encouraging fat storage in your body. This can even cause insulin resistance, storage of fat in the liver, and diabetes.

Additionally, a lack of sleep upsets the balance of leptin and ghrelin. Leptin is responsible for telling you when you are full, which means you feel hungry even when you are not. Ghrelin stimulates hunger and reduces hormones in excess, and a lack of sleep encourages its production.

Additionally, not getting enough sleep can affect the frontal lobe, which is responsible for decision making. This can leave you more susceptible to poor dieting choices because it becomes increasingly hard to resist the temptation.

Mistake #17: You Aren't Choosing the Right Diet for Your Body

One of the problems with fad diets is that they treat everyone as the same rather than as the individual that they are. For example, some people respond well to a reduced-calorie diet, while others cut out fat and are successful. However, not everyone's body is built the same way. For some people, low-carbohydrate diets are the best option.

One variation of low-carb diets is a Ketogenic diet, where you increase protein and fat intake while reducing carbohydrates almost completely. Some studies have shown that in the short term, these diets cause as much as two to three times the amount of weight loss as a typical low-fat diet. Additionally, low-carb diets can improve good cholesterol levels, manage blood sugar, and improve triglycerides.

Ideally, the diet you choose should reflect factors like your metabolism and what your problem areas are. This will help you find the diet that is most effective. Additionally, keep in mind that many diets have additional health benefits, not just weight loss. Consider what will help you the most, and adjust as needed until you see the results that you want.

Finally, be patient with the results. You often cannot tell if a diet is working for several weeks because of the numerous factors that cause weight to fluctuate.

Mistake #18: You Are Drinking Too Much

It is not always the food that we are putting in our bodies that is the problem when it comes to weight loss. Even supposedly healthy drinks, such as vitamin beverages and juices, are high in sugar, which can contribute to an increased caloric intake. This is problematic because beverages are not filling. This means that you are taking in these extra carbohydrates and still craving food. These drinks are okay in moderation, but too much can be problematic.

The amount of water you drink can also affect how much weight you are gaining or losing. When you drink water, it has been proven that the number of calories you burn can be boosted for the next hour and a half by an impressive 24% to 30%. Another study showed that drinking about two cups (17 ounces) of water about half an hour prior to a meal increased weight loss by 44%. This means that if you are dieting, drinking water can drastically boost the results you are seeing.

Alcohol can be another problem beverage for weight loss. Beers and some types of sugary liquors have high sugar content that can add unnecessary calories. Additionally, most alcohols contain seven calories per gram of liquid. This does not mean that you have to quit completely, but try to drink only moderate amounts of alcohol. You should also stick to vodka and other spirits, mixed with a beverage that does not have calories.

Mistake #19: You Are Trying to Lose Too Much Too Fast

People who are trying to lose weight often want to see results fast. The problem with this is that rapid weight loss is not healthy for the body. It is also nearly impossible to maintain if you go back to a normal or less intense diet and exercise regimen.

The best way to lose weight is gradually. The people who are most effective at maintaining their weight loss may lose just 1 to 2 pounds of weight each week or less.

Something else to keep in mind regarding expectations is that there are external factors that can influence weight gain. For example, having conditions like PCOS, diabetes, hyperthyroidism, or sleep apnea can cause weight gain. There are also many medications for treating different conditions that can cause the person taking them to gain weight. If you believe that an underlying condition or a medication may be the root of your struggles in losing weight, consult with your physician about the best route for you to take.

Mistake #20: Your Body Needs a Break

Constant dieting is not healthy. Additionally, when you diet for a long period of time, you may find that you start gaining back weight the moment you decide to try and manage your weight rather than losing it. This has a lot to do with the body's set point, which can be lowered—but must be lowered gradually to be effective.

Sometimes, the best thing to do when you plateau with weight loss is not to fight back harder by reducing calories more or increasing your workout. Instead, try taking a break from weight loss, and work to maintain that weight. By maintaining a lower weight, you will help adjust your body's weight set point.

Ideally, you should take a break and try to maintain that lower weight for one to two months before starting another diet and exercise regimen. During this time, make sure you are getting plenty of sleep and still working to build lean muscle. By doing this, you are encouraging your overall health and ensuring that you maintain your weight loss instead of gaining it back, as many people do.

Conclusion

When you are trying to lose weight, there are many factors fighting against you. Fortunately, knowledge is half the battle when it comes to understanding your body and why you may not be losing weight. Take a good look at your weight loss efforts, and compare them against the information you have read so far. Chances are you will find the reason or reasons why you have not been successful.

The good news is that it is never too late to start working toward a healthier, happier, and fitter you. Take your new knowledge, and use it to help you lose weight in a way that works. Learn to listen to your body—you can often tell by the way that it feels what it needs.

Thank you, and remember to share how well these weight loss tips work for you. You can do that by writing a review in your Amazon account under Your Orders.

Thank you,

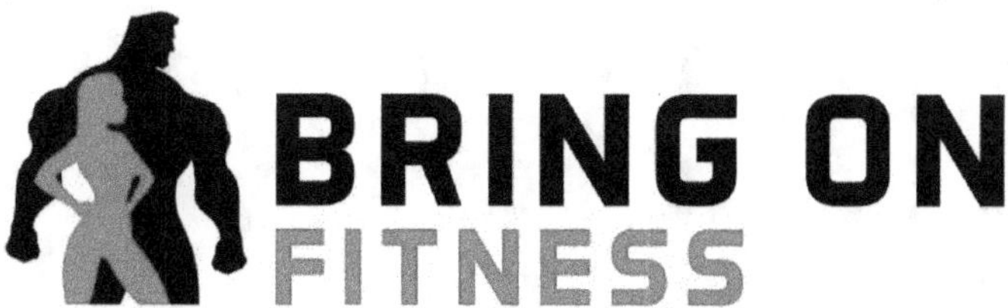

References

http://www.fitnessforweightloss.com/diet-and-weight-loss-statistics/

https://www.cnn.com/2016/01/28/health/weight-loss-exercise-plateau/index.html

https://www.nytimes.com/2016/05/08/opinion/sunday/why-you-cant-lose-weight-on-a-diet.html

http://www.findingbalance.com/articles/understanding-hunger-and-fullness-cues/

https://www.healthline.com/nutrition/how-protein-can-help-you-lose-weight

https://www.healthline.com/nutrition/20-reasons-you-are-not-losing-weight#section3

https://www.cbsnews.com/news/can-diet-soda-make-you-gain-weight/

https://www.shape.com/lifestyle/mind-and-body/why-sleep-no-1-most-important-thing-better-body